COMPLETE GUIDE TO LIVER DISEASE

Comprehensive Overview Of Symptoms, Causes, Diagnosis, Treatments, Nutrition, And Preventive Strategies For Optimal Hepatic Health

DEHART HAIRSTON

© [DEHART HAIRSTON], [2024]

All rights reserved. No part of this publication may be reproduced, distributed, or transmitted in any form or by any means, including photocopying, recording, or other electronic or mechanical methods, without the prior written permission of the publisher, except in the case of brief quotations embodied in critical reviews and certain other noncommercial uses permitted by copyright law.

DISCLAIMER

This book's content is only intended for general informative purposes. At the time of writing, the author has taken every precaution to guarantee that the material is correct and current. Nevertheless, the author disclaims all explicit and implicit representations and guarantees about the availability, appropriateness, correctness, completeness, and usefulness of the material on these pages.

Since the author is not a licensed medical practitioner, the material in this book shouldn't be interpreted as medical advice. Before making any modifications to their diet, exercise regimen, or medical treatment, readers are urged to speak with a licensed healthcare provider.

Moreover, the author has no connection to any of the businesses, organizations, or people that are discussed in this book. Any mentions of goods, services, businesses, or people are purely informative and do not indicate endorsement or suggestion.

This book's content is entirely dependent on the author's expertise, study, and comprehension of the topic. Despite having taken reasonable care to offer correct information, the author disclaims all liability for any mistakes or omissions in the material as well as for any losses, harm, or damages resulting from using the information.

It is recommended that readers use their own judgment and discretion when applying the knowledge in this book to their own situations. The use or implementation of any material in this book may result in unfavorable repercussions, directly or indirectly, for which the author assumes no liability.

By reading this book, you agree to release and hold the author harmless from any claims, losses, liabilities, costs, or expenditures resulting from or related to the use of the information you get from it.

Table of Contents

CHAPTER 1 13
Understanding The Liver 13
Introduction To The Liver And Its Functions 13
Importance Of A Healthy Liver 14
Common Liver Diseases And Their Impact 16
1. Fatty Liver Disease: 16
3. Liver Cirrhosis: 17

CHAPTER 2 19
Anatomy Of The Liver 19
Structure And Location Of The Liver 19
Overview Of Liver Lobes And Segments 20
Blood Supply And Bile Production 21

CHAPTER 3 23
Causes Of Liver Disease 23
Explanation Of Liver Disease Etiology 23
Risk Factors Such As Alcohol, Viruses, And Genetics 25
Lifestyle Factors Contributing To Liver Health 26

CHAPTER 4 29
Types Of Liver Diseases 29
Hepatitis (A, B, C) 29

Hepatitis A: 29
Hepatitis B: 30
Hepatitis C: 30
Cirrhosis 31
Fatty Liver Disease 33
Hepatic Cancer 35

CHAPTER 5 39
Symptoms And Diagnosis 39
Recognizing Symptoms Of Liver Disease 39
Diagnostic Tests And Procedures 40
Blood Tests 41
Imaging Studies (Ultrasound, Mri, Ct Scan) 42
Liver Biopsy 43

CHAPTER 6 45
Treatment Options 45
Medical Interventions 45
   Drugs for Different Liver Illnesses: 45
   Modifications in Lifestyle: 46
Surgical Techniques 48
   Transplantation of the liver: 48
   Resection via Surgery: 49

CHAPTER 7 53
Managing Liver Disease 53
Medication Adherence 53
Dietary Considerations 55
Avoiding Alcohol And Harmful Substances 57

CHAPTER 8 59
Support And Resources 59
Counseling Services For Patients And Caregivers . 59
Reliable Sources For Liver Disease Information ... 61

CHAPTER 9 65
Preventing Liver Disease 65
Prevention Strategies For Maintaining Liver Health
.... 65

- 2. Moderate Alcohol drinking: 65
- 3. Frequent Exercise: 66
- 4. Avoiding Hazardous Substances: 66
- 5. Adopt Safe Sexual Behavior: 66
- 6. Keep Your Weight in Check: 67
- 7. Keep Yourself Hydrated: 67
- 8. Get Regular Check-ups: 67

Vaccinations For Hepatitis Viruses 68

- 1. Hepatitis B vaccination: ... 68
- 2. Hepatitis A Vaccine: ... 69
- 3. Combination vaccines: ... 69
- 4. Immunization Schedule: ... 70
- 5. Vaccine Safety: ... 70
- 7. Access to Vaccines: ... 71

Screening Recommendations For At-Risk Individuals ... 72

- 1. Hepatitis B Screening: ... 72
- 2. Hepatitis C Screening: ... 73
- 3. Tests for Liver Function: ... 73
- 4. Imaging Studies: ... 74
- 5. Fibrosis Assessment: ... 74
- 6. Screening Frequency: ... 75

CHAPTER 10 ... 77

Living With Liver Disease ... 77

Coping Mechanisms For Managing Chronic Liver Conditions ... 77

Maintaining Quality Of Life While Living With Liver Disease ... 79

Hope For The Future: Advances In Liver Disease Research And Treatment ... 82

CONCLUSION 85
THE END 88

ABOUT THE BOOK

"Liver Disease" is more than simply a book; it's a vital resource for understanding, treating, and avoiding liver diseases. The liver is an essential organ that performs several tasks that are critical to our general health and well-being. Starting with the fundamentals in Chapter 1, readers will understand the importance of a healthy liver and become familiar with common liver illnesses and their implications. This book functions as a thorough roadmap.

The liver's complex architecture is explored in detail in Chapter 2, along with information on its location, structure, and vital roles like bile generation and blood supply. Comprehending the structure of the liver is essential to appreciating the complexity of liver illnesses covered in later chapters.

The causes of liver illness are explained in detail in Chapter 3, covering everything from genetic predispositions to lifestyle decisions, so that readers are fully aware of the variables that might impact liver health. In the meanwhile, Chapter 4 provides readers with a thorough review of a range of liver illnesses, including hepatitis and liver cancer, along with information on their symptoms, course, and available treatments.

Not content to stop at diagnosis and therapy, the book also explores management techniques for liver disease (Chapter 7), offering a comprehensive approach that includes dietary considerations, lifestyle modifications, and drug adherence. Furthermore, it provides readers with a lifeline in Chapter 8 by putting them in touch with reputable resources, counseling services, and support groups for overcoming the difficulties associated with liver illness.

But the most important part is probably found in Chapter 9, which lays out preventative techniques. Equipped with information on immunizations, screening suggestions, and lifestyle adjustments, readers may proactively protect their liver health.

In conclusion, Chapter 10 offers a glimmer of hope by highlighting coping strategies and developments in the study and treatment of liver disease. "Liver Disease" equips readers with knowledge and tools, making it a valuable resource for anybody trying to comprehend, treat, and eventually overcome liver conditions.

CHAPTER 1

Understanding The Liver

Introduction To The Liver And Its Functions

The liver, also known as the body's chemical factory, is a powerful organ. It is located in the upper right section of the abdomen and is essential to preserving general health and well-being. What does the liver accomplish, though? Let's examine how it works.

The liver is primarily in charge of processing the nutrients in the food we eat. The break down proteins, lipids, and carbs, either turning them into energy or storing them for later. The liver also helps in detoxification by removing toxins, alcohol, and other dangerous chemicals from the circulation.

The liver generates bile, a digestive fluid necessary for the small intestine to break down lipids, in addition to metabolism and cleansing. This procedure makes it easier for nutrients to be properly absorbed and digested. In addition, the liver produces the proteins required for immunological response, blood coagulation, and the preservation of the body's fluid balance.

The liver is essentially a multitasking wonder that carries out a multitude of key tasks that are essential to our overall health and well-being.

Importance Of A Healthy Liver

Having a healthy liver is essential for well-being given its critical role in preserving general health. Our internal environment is maintained in balance when the liver is operating at its best, which makes sure that vital activities go without a hitch.

Regrettably, the liver may suffer harm from several conditions, such as heavy alcohol use, viral infections (like hepatitis), obesity, and several drugs. The liver's many activities are hampered when it is damaged, which may result in a variety of health problems.

If left untreated, liver illnesses such as cirrhosis, liver cancer, and fatty liver disease may have catastrophic effects. Therefore, it's critical to have a healthy lifestyle and develop behaviors that support liver health. This entails abstaining from dangerous behaviors including intravenous drug use, exercising often, eating a balanced diet full of fruits, vegetables, and whole grains, and minimizing alcohol use.

Frequent visits to a healthcare professional may also help in the early diagnosis and treatment of liver problems, which may limit additional harm and improve results. By placing a high priority on liver health, people may protect their general health and well-being.

Common Liver Diseases And Their Impact

A wide range of disorders are included in the term "liver diseases," each having unique origins, signs, and effects. Among the most prevalent liver conditions are:

1. Fatty Liver Disease: This illness is brought on by the buildup of extra fat in the liver, which is often brought on by obesity, insulin resistance, or heavy alcohol use. Over time, non-alcoholic steatohepatitis (NASH), a more severe type of fatty liver disease, may induce inflammation and damage to the liver.

2. Hepatitis is an infection of the liver that may be brought on by viruses (hepatitis A, B, C, etc.), excessive alcohol usage, autoimmune diseases, certain drugs, and toxins. If chronic hepatitis is not properly treated, it might result in liver cancer or cirrhosis.

3. Liver Cirrhosis: The hallmark of cirrhosis is the scarring of liver tissue, which is often brought on by chronic inflammation and injury to the liver. Ascites, or an accumulation of fluid in the abdomen, portal hypertension, and hepatic encephalopathy—brain dysfunction brought on by liver failure—are among the consequences that may result from this scarring, which also affects liver function.

4. Hepatocellular carcinoma, another name for primary liver cancer, is a disease that starts in the liver and is often linked to cirrhosis or long-term hepatitis B or C infection. When cancer from another region of the body spreads (metastasizes) to the liver, it results in secondary liver cancer.

The quality of life and general health of a person might be greatly impacted by certain liver illnesses. While symptoms might vary, some common ones include exhaustion, nausea, vomiting, stomach discomfort and swelling, jaundice (yellowing of the skin and eyes), and unexplained weight loss. To successfully manage liver illnesses and minimize their influence on overall health, early identification and management are essential.

CHAPTER 2

Anatomy Of The Liver

Structure And Location Of The Liver

Located beneath the rib cage on the right side of the abdomen, the liver is an essential organ often referred to as the body's chemical factory. Its well-planned location makes it simple to access blood exiting the digestive system. The liver is a wedge-shaped, reddish-brown organ with a rubbery feel that weighs around three pounds in adults. Although it might vary somewhat in size from person to person, it usually measures around the same as a football.

The liver is separated into two major lobes, the smaller left lobe and the larger right lobe. Each part of the liver has its blood supply and function. The ability to precisely target particular parts of the liver during medical procedures like operations or targeted therapies is made possible by this segmentation. In addition, the liver's structure and form are preserved by a thin, fibrous coating known as Glisson's capsule.

Overview Of Liver Lobes And Segments

The segments and lobes of the liver are essential to its operation. The right lobe makes up around two-thirds of the liver's mass since it is heavier and bigger than the left lobe. The right anterior and right posterior parts make up its further division. On the other hand, the left lobe is separated into the left medial and left lateral portions; it is smaller but just as significant. These sections aren't simply random splits; they match certain bile ducts and blood veins, which helps with surgical techniques and comprehension of liver function.

To accurately target sick or damaged parts while protecting good tissue, surgeons must have a thorough understanding of these segments before performing liver procedures. This accuracy shortens healing periods and reduces problems. Each segment also has its blood supply, so even if one is damaged, the others may still operate, although at a diminished capacity. This redundancy is evidence of the liver's extraordinary regeneration ability and durability.

Blood Supply And Bile Production

The liver's diverse range of activities depends on its unique dual blood supply. The hepatic artery, which transports blood from the heart that is high in oxygen, provides around 25% of the blood supply. The remaining 75% travels from the digestive system to the portal vein, which carries blood that is rich in nutrients. Blood that is both nutrient-rich and oxygenated gives the liver the energy it needs to perform a wide range of metabolic processes, such as protein synthesis, detoxification, and glycogen storage.

The liver's complex system of bile ducts is where bile generation takes place, which is another essential function of the liver. The liver cells, or hepatocytes, produce bile, a greenish-yellow fluid, which is then moved via a network of bile ducts and either retained in the gallbladder or discharged straight into the small intestine. Bile facilitates fat absorption in the colon by emulsifying them, which helps indigestion. Bile also acts as a means of the body's excretion of waste materials, including cholesterol and bilirubin.

To fully appreciate the liver's function in preserving general health, one must have a basic understanding of its architecture, which includes knowledge of its lobes, segments, blood supply, and bile generation.

CHAPTER 3

Causes Of Liver Disease

Explanation Of Liver Disease Etiology

The fundamental reasons for liver disease are known as the etiology, and they are many and varied. It is essential to comprehend these factors to manage and prevent liver-related disorders properly. Numerous variables, such as viral infections, alcohol misuse, genetic predispositions, autoimmune illnesses, and metabolic imbalances, may result in liver diseases.

Viral hepatitis, which is caused by the hepatitis A, B, C, D, and E viruses, is one of the main causes of liver disease. Viral hepatitis may cause either acute or chronic liver inflammation, which can develop into more serious diseases including cirrhosis or liver cancer.

If treatment is not received, hepatitis B and C are especially well-known for their propensity to result in chronic infection and permanent liver damage.

Liver disease is also significantly influenced by alcohol intake. Alcoholic liver disease (ALD) is a group of disorders that includes fatty liver, alcoholic hepatitis, and cirrhosis. Chronic alcohol misuse may cause ALD. Overindulgence in alcohol gradually overpowers the liver's capacity to process alcohol, resulting in damage, inflammation, and compromised liver function.

The prevalence of non-alcoholic fatty liver disease (NAFLD) is rising, and it's often linked to metabolic syndrome, obesity, and insulin resistance. The term "NAFLD" refers to a group of illnesses marked by an overabundance of fat accumulating in the liver, which may lead to cirrhosis, fibrosis, and inflammation. Obesity, sedentary activity, and poor nutrition are examples of lifestyle variables that greatly contribute to the onset and progression of NAFLD.

Risk Factors Such As Alcohol, Viruses, And Genetics

The chance of having liver disease is increased by several risk factors, which emphasizes the need for early detection and prevention. People may take proactive measures to preserve their liver and make educated choices about their health by being aware of these risk factors.

Drinking alcohol is one of the main risk factors for liver disease, and heavy and prolonged drinking increases the chance of getting ALD. The degree of liver damage is influenced by the quantity and duration of alcohol intake, underscoring the need for moderation and appropriate drinking practices.

There is a considerable danger associated with viral hepatitis, especially hepatitis B and C, which, if ignored, may cause chronic infection and progressive liver damage. The need for immunization, safe sex practices, and prenatal care is underscored by the prevalent mechanisms of transmission of hepatitis, which include unsafe injecting behaviors, unprotected sexual activity, and vertical transmission from mother to child.

Hepatic disease susceptibility is also influenced by genetic factors. A person may be more susceptible to diseases that impair liver function and raise the risk of liver damage, such as hemochromatosis, Wilson's disease, or alpha-1 antitrypsin deficiency, due to certain genetic mutations or variations.

Lifestyle Factors Contributing To Liver Health

Adopting lifestyle practices that promote normal liver function and reduce the risk of liver disease is essential to maintaining liver health.

Several important lifestyle choices may both prevent or slow the development of diseases connected to the liver.

For liver health, a diet that is both balanced and nutrient-dense is crucial, giving the body the nutrients it needs while reducing the consumption of fats, sweets, and processed foods. A diet high in fruits, vegetables, whole grains, lean meats, and healthy fats promotes liver health and protects against diseases such as nonalcoholic fatty liver disease (NAFLD) and liver disease linked to obesity.

Frequent exercise is essential for liver health because it helps control weight, enhances insulin sensitivity, and lowers inflammation. A weekly regimen that includes strength training, flexibility exercises, and aerobic exercise may help maintain a healthy weight and lower the risk of metabolic syndrome and non-alcoholic fatty liver disease (NAFLD).

Maintaining liver health and avoiding alcohol-related liver disease require reducing or eliminating alcohol use. To reduce the risk of liver damage, people should consume alcohol in moderation and according to prescribed standards.

The risk of liver damage may be decreased by avoiding exposure to hepatotoxic substances and by adopting safe practices, such as wearing protective gear while handling chemicals or prescription drugs. In addition, liver health may be safeguarded by engaging in safe sexual behavior, receiving a hepatitis vaccination, and refraining from sharing sanitary products or needles.

People may lower their risk of liver disease and maintain liver health by leading a healthy lifestyle that includes a balanced diet, frequent exercise, reduction in alcohol intake, and safe behaviors. Maintaining the liver in good condition is crucial for general health and lifespan.

CHAPTER 4

Types Of Liver Diseases

Hepatitis (A, B, C)

The word "hepatitis," which is often used but not usually understood, describes an inflammation of the liver. Hepatitis A, B, and C are the most prevalent forms, however there are others as well. Let's dissect them.

Hepatitis A: Food or water contamination is the typical source of this kind of infection. It's often linked to inadequate hygiene or sanitation. Fatigue, nausea, stomach discomfort, and jaundice (yellowing of the skin and eyes) are possible symptoms. Fortunately, there is a vaccination that may prevent Hepatitis A, and most survivors completely recover without developing long-term liver damage.

Hepatitis B: Hepatitis B is spread via body fluids such as blood, semen, or saliva, in contrast to Hepatitis A. It may either develop chronic and cause long-term liver issues, or it can be acute, lasting just a short while before clearing up on its own. Hepatitis A symptoms are the same, albeit they might be more severe. Hepatitis B vaccination is also an option, and it is especially important for those who are at risk, including healthcare professionals or those who have many sexual partners.

Hepatitis C: Contact with contaminated blood is the main way that hepatitis C is transmitted. The symptoms of Hepatitis C might take years or even decades to manifest in many cases. Serious liver damage, including cirrhosis and liver cancer, may result from this insidious development. Hepatitis C cannot be prevented, although it may be managed with antiviral drugs. For therapy to be effective and problems to be avoided, early identification is essential.

Comprehending the distinctions among various varieties of Hepatitis is essential for both prevention and treatment. A few key tactics to lower the chance of contracting Hepatitis include vaccination, safe sex practices, not sharing needles, and proper cleanliness.

Cirrhosis

The disease known as cirrhosis causes scar tissue to progressively replace good liver tissue, therefore compromising liver function. It often arises from persistent drinking, hepatitis B or C infection, non-alcoholic fatty liver disease, or other disorders that cause long-term liver damage. Cirrhosis may take years to grow, and symptoms might not show up until serious harm has been done.

Fatigue, weakness, easy bruising or bleeding, jaundice, and swelling in the belly and legs are common signs of cirrhosis. As the illness progresses, side effects include ascites (a buildup of fluid in the abdomen), portal hypertension (high blood pressure in the liver), and hepatic encephalopathy (impaired brain function brought on by liver failure).

Treating the underlying cause of cirrhosis—be it quitting drinking, taking antiviral medication for Hepatitis infections, or making lifestyle adjustments to control fatty liver disease—is essential to managing the condition. The goals of treatment are to manage problems, stop more liver damage, and enhance quality of life. When liver damage is severe and the patient has advanced cirrhosis, liver transplantation may be required.

To improve outcomes and decrease the course of cirrhosis, early detection and management are essential. A treatment plan that is adhered to and routine medical monitoring may help people with cirrhosis live longer, healthier lives.

Fatty Liver Disease

As the name implies, fatty liver disease is caused by an abnormal accumulation of fat in the liver. Alcoholic fatty liver disease (AFLD) and non-alcoholic fatty liver disease (NAFLD) are the two primary forms.

Alcoholic Fatty Liver Disease (AFLD): Overindulgence in alcohol over time leads to the development of AFLD. Alcohol is metabolized by the liver, but too much of it may overload it and cause inflammation and fat storage. If drinking persists, AFLD may develop into more serious illnesses such as cirrhosis and alcoholic hepatitis.

Fatty liver disease (NAFLD) that is not associated with alcohol use is more prevalent. Obesity, insulin resistance, type 2 diabetes, elevated cholesterol, and metabolic syndrome are all closely linked to it. Simple fatty liver disease (steatosis) and non-alcoholic steatohepatitis (NASH), which causes inflammation in the liver and may lead to cirrhosis and liver cancer, are the two forms of NAFLD.

At first, fatty liver disease symptoms may not be very noticeable, but as the illness worsens, people may start to feel tired and have pain in their abdomens as well as an enlarged liver. To evaluate liver function and rule out other disorders, imaging investigations and blood tests are often used in the diagnosis process.

The mainstay of treatment for fatty liver disease is changing one's lifestyle to include things like drinking less alcohol, losing weight, exercising often, and eating a nutritious diet. It's also critical to manage underlying illnesses like diabetes and high cholesterol. Medication may be used in more severe situations to lessen liver inflammation and stop more liver damage.

For those with fatty liver disease, routine medical monitoring is crucial to determining the course of the condition and reducing consequences. Many patients with fatty liver disease may prevent or halt the illness's course and improve their liver function with early intervention and lifestyle modifications.

Hepatic Cancer

Hepatocellular carcinoma (HCC), another name for liver cancer, may occur as a primary cancer that starts in the liver or as a secondary cancer that spreads to other regions of the body. Liver cancer risk is increased by chronic liver illnesses such as cirrhosis, fatty liver disease, and chronic Hepatitis B or C infections.

Abdominal discomfort, edema, jaundice, and unexplained weight loss are all possible signs of liver cancer. However, liver cancer may not exhibit any signs in its early stages, which makes early identification difficult.

Imaging studies including ultrasounds, CT scans, and MRIs are often used in conjunction with blood tests to measure tumor markers and liver function to make a diagnosis. Depending on the disease's stage, liver cancer may be treated with surgery, chemotherapy, radiation treatment, targeted therapy, or liver transplantation.

Reducing risk factors for liver cancer includes abstaining from excessive alcohol use, receiving the Hepatitis B vaccine, keeping a healthy weight, and taking care of ongoing liver diseases. In high-risk patients, such as those with cirrhosis, routine screening for liver cancer may aid in the early detection of tumors when therapy is most successful.

In general, early identification, intervention, and treatment of liver disorders depend on an awareness of the many forms of liver diseases, their symptoms, and their course. People may safeguard their liver health and lower their chance of consequences from liver illnesses by leading healthy lifestyles, getting medical attention when necessary, and adhering to treatment guidelines.

CHAPTER 5

Symptoms And Diagnosis

Recognizing Symptoms Of Liver Disease

A quick diagnosis and course of therapy for liver illness depends on the recognition of its symptoms, which may present in a variety of ways. Certain symptoms may be more noticeable and suggestive of underlying liver disorders, while others may be more subdued or readily confused for other medical conditions.

Jaundice, which is characterized by yellowing of the skin and eyes, is one of the most prevalent indications of liver illness. This happens when the waste substance bilirubin, which is created when old red blood cells degrade, cannot be properly processed by the liver. Additional symptoms might include edema and soreness in the abdomen, especially around the liver, which is situated in the upper right section of the abdomen. Hepatic dysfunction may also be indicated by weakness, exhaustion, and inexplicable weight reduction.

Furthermore, dark urine and changes in bowel patterns, such as pale or clay-colored stools, may occur in liver disease patients. It's crucial to remember that not every person with liver disease will experience every single one of these symptoms and that the degree and mix of symptoms might change based on the underlying reason and stage of the illness.

Diagnostic Tests And Procedures

A physical examination, a review of the patient's medical history, and several diagnostic tests and procedures are usually used to diagnose liver disease. These assist medical professionals in evaluating liver function, figuring out the disease's underlying etiology, and estimating the degree of liver damage.

Blood Tests

Blood tests are often used to assess liver health and find anomalies in liver enzyme levels and other chemicals that may indicate damage or malfunction to the liver. The liver function panel, which examines levels of enzymes including alanine aminotransferase (ALT), aspartate aminotransferase (AST), alkaline phosphatase (ALP), and bilirubin, is one of the main blood tests used in the assessment of liver disease. Increased concentrations of these enzymes may be a sign of injury, inflammation, or poor liver function.

Blood tests may be used to evaluate various parameters, such as clotting factors, albumin levels, and the presence of certain antibodies or viral indicators linked to certain liver illnesses, including hepatitis B or C, in addition to liver function tests.

Imaging Studies (Ultrasound, Mri, Ct Scan)

Imaging tests are essential for the diagnosis and assessment of liver disease. When evaluating the liver and associated tissues, ultrasound is often the first imaging modality to be employed. It may provide important details on the size, texture, and structure of the liver as well as if any anomalies such as tumors, cysts, or fatty infiltration are present.

Magnetic resonance imaging (MRI) or computed tomography (CT) scans may be carried out in situations when more imaging is necessary or when more information is required. These imaging modalities may distinguish between distinct liver disorders, such as cirrhosis, fatty liver disease, or liver malignancies, and provide comprehensive cross-sectional pictures of the liver.

Liver Biopsy

A liver biopsy could be advised in certain circumstances to collect a tissue sample for a thorough microscopic inspection. A liver biopsy involves the use of a needle guided by ultrasound or CT imaging to extract a tiny sample of liver tissue. A pathologist then examines the sample to look for indications of infection, cancer, fibrosis, inflammation, or fatty infiltration.

Liver biopsies are seen to be the gold standard for identifying certain liver disorders and may provide important data that helps influence therapy choices. But since it's an intrusive surgery, there's a little chance of problems including bleeding and infection.

CHAPTER 6

Treatment Options

Medical Interventions

Drugs for Different Liver Illnesses:

Medication is an essential part of treating liver illnesses since it helps to manage symptoms, slow down the disease's course, and in some cases even reverse the condition. The particular liver disease that a person is dealing with determines the kind of medicine that is administered. For example, antiviral drugs are often used to inhibit the virus's reproduction and lessen liver inflammation in instances of viral hepatitis.

Corticosteroids are another family of drugs that are often used to treat liver disease. These are often recommended to lower inflammation in illnesses like autoimmune hepatitis, a disease in which the immune system of the body unintentionally targets the liver.

Additionally, chelating drugs like penicillamine or trientine may assist in eliminating excess copper in Wilson's disease, while pharmaceuticals like ursodeoxycholic acid (UDCA) may be administered to enhance bile flow in situations like primary biliary cholangitis.

Patients with liver problems must follow their doctors recommended drug schedule to the letter. Medication mistakes or sudden stops might have dangerous repercussions and make the illness worse.

Modifications in Lifestyle:

Modifications to lifestyle are important in controlling liver illnesses in addition to medicine. Adopting a nutritious diet is among the most significant lifestyle improvements that people can undertake.

Consuming a diet high in fruits, vegetables, healthy grains, and lean meats may improve general health and liver function. In addition, because diets rich in saturated fats and alcohol may aggravate liver damage, it's critical to restrict alcohol intake.

Exercise regularly is another essential part of changing one's lifestyle to control liver disease. Engaging in physical exercise lowers the chance of developing fatty liver disease, improves general cardiovascular health, and helps maintain a healthy weight. A small amount of activity, like swimming or brisk walking, may have a significant positive impact on liver function.

Furthermore, liver function must be preserved by limiting exposure to poisons and dangerous chemicals. This entails refraining from using illegal drugs and, to the greatest extent feasible, reducing one's exposure to chemicals and pollutants in the environment.

Surgical Techniques

Transplantation of the liver:

If a person has liver failure or severe liver disease, a liver transplant can be their last chance for long-term life. A healthy liver from a dead or living donor is used to replace the damaged liver during a liver transplant. For people suffering from acute liver failure, liver cancer, or end-stage liver disease, this operation may be life-saving.

Hepatologists, transplant surgeons, nurses, social workers, and other multidisciplinary healthcare personnel must carefully assess and coordinate the difficult process of liver transplant surgery. A thorough pre-transplant examination is required of patients receiving liver transplants to determine their eligibility and appropriateness for the surgery.

To avoid organ rejection after a liver transplant, patients will need to take immunosuppressive drugs for the rest of their lives. These drugs lessen the immune system's reaction to the liver transplant, which lowers the chance of rejection but raises the risk of infection. It's crucial to schedule routine follow-up visits with medical professionals to check for problems or indications of rejection and to change prescription doses as necessary.

Resection via Surgery:

Surgical resection may be advised when liver tumors are circumscribed and amenable to removal by surgery. The surgery involves removing the tumor-containing part of the liver while leaving the healthy liver tissue intact. For benign liver lesions like hepatic adenomas or liver cancer, surgical excision is often necessary.

The size and location of the tumor, the patient's general health, and the degree of liver function are some of the variables that affect the outcome of surgical excision. Patients will be thoroughly evaluated, including imaging scans and blood tests, before surgery to determine if they are candidates for the treatment.

Patients usually go through a recuperation phase after surgical resection, during which time they are constantly watched for any indications of problems, such as bleeding or infection. To guarantee the best possible healing and recovery, patients must adhere to their doctor's post-operative recommendations, which may include dietary adjustments, limits on physical activity, and medication management.

To sum up, many different liver disease treatment choices may be customized to meet the unique demands and circumstances of each patient. The objective is to control symptoms, improve liver function, and eventually improve quality of life, whether using surgical treatments like liver transplantation and surgical resection or pharmacological therapies like medication and lifestyle modifications.

CHAPTER 7

Managing Liver Disease

Medication Adherence

Treatment adherence is crucial for the efficient management of liver disease. Prescription drugs from medical professionals are essential for managing symptoms, delaying the course of the illness, and enhancing liver function in general. However, it's essential to strictly adhere to the recommended dose and regimen for these drugs to function at their best.

When it comes to taking liver disease drugs, consistency is essential. Missing doses or deviating from the recommended regimen might worsen symptoms and hurt liver function. It's critical to comprehend the role that each drug plays in helping to manage the illness.

Medication adherence may be maintained by establishing a routine. Using smartphone applications, pillbox organization, or setting reminders may help ensure that prescriptions are taken on time. Furthermore, maintaining a drug notebook to record dosages and any adverse effects may provide medical professionals with important information to modify therapy as necessary.

Having open lines of contact with medical professionals is essential for resolving any issues or problems with drug adherence. They may provide assistance, direction, and substitute remedies if certain drugs cause problems or adverse reactions. Recalling that taking medicine as prescribed is essential for treating hepatic illness might spur people to stick to their treatment regimen.

Dietary Considerations

To manage liver disease and promote liver health, a proper diet is essential. A balanced diet may lessen symptoms, promote general health, and lessen the strain on the liver. For those with liver illness, knowing which foods to include and which to avoid is crucial.

For the health of the liver, a diet high in fruits, vegetables, whole grains, and lean meats is recommended. These foods include vital nutrients, fiber, and antioxidants that support the body's detoxification, metabolic, and digestive processes. Drinking plenty of water and herbal teas can also aid in the removal of toxins from the body and maintain the liver's moisture levels.

Reducing the consumption of certain foods and substances is essential for the management of liver disease. Fried, high-fat, and processed meals may put a burden on the liver and aggravate fatty liver disease and inflammation. In a similar vein, consuming too much sugar and salt might impair liver function and make symptoms worse.

For those who have liver disease, alcohol intake should be tightly controlled or avoided since it might worsen the condition. Alcohol may damage the liver even in tiny doses, thus it's important to either fully abstain from alcohol or abide by the doctor's instructions.

A trained dietitian or nutritionist may provide individualized nutritional advice based on each person's requirements and preferences. They may assist with meal planning, provide advice on regulating portion sizes, and provide techniques for juggling social obligations with nutritional requirements.

Avoiding Alcohol And Harmful Substances

A vital component of controlling hepatic illness is abstaining from alcohol and other toxic drugs, which may worsen symptoms and hasten the disease's advancement. Due to its ability to induce cirrhosis, fatty liver disease, inflammation, and liver failure, alcohol is very harmful to the health of the liver.

For those with liver illness, total abstinence from alcohol is advised, irrespective of the severity or underlying reason. Alcohol use, even in small doses, may have a significant impact on liver health and general well-being. Alcohol intake has concerns that should be understood, and liver health should come first.

The health of the liver may also be endangered by certain prescription pharmaceuticals, recreational drugs, and environmental pollutants in addition to alcohol. Before beginning any new supplement regimen or prescription, it is important to speak with your doctor to be sure it is safe for those with liver disease.

Preserving liver health requires avoiding exposure to hazardous chemicals both at home and at work. Chemicals, solvents, and heavy metals are examples of workplace dangers that may harm the liver and raise the risk of liver disease. Liver damage may be avoided and exposure can be reduced by taking the appropriate safety measures, such as donning protective clothing and adhering to safety procedures.

Promoting liver health and avoiding liver disease requires educating oneself and other people about the risks associated with alcohol use and other toxic drugs.

CHAPTER 8

Support And Resources

Counseling Services For Patients And Caregivers

Counseling services are a vital source of support for liver disease patients and their carers. Stress, anxiety, despair, and other emotional difficulties may result from having a chronic disease, which can hurt mental health. To discuss these psychological issues and create coping mechanisms, professional therapy offers a private, secure setting.

Counseling may assist patients in navigating the emotional ups and downs associated with diagnosis, treatment, and recovery. It offers a safe space for people to share their worries, annoyances, and concerns while picking up useful coping skills. Counselors with experience managing chronic illnesses may provide individualized advice based on the requirements of each client.

Counseling services are also very beneficial to caregivers since caring for a loved one with liver disease often results in high levels of stress and exhaustion. Counseling sessions may support caregivers in prioritizing self-care above other obligations, setting boundaries, and managing their emotions. Counselors may also provide helpful advice on how to improve resilience, problem-solving, and communication in the caregiver-patient relationship.

Additionally, family therapy sessions may be included in counseling services, giving patients and their loved ones the chance to work through interpersonal issues, strengthen bonds, and promote understanding. Patients who include their family members in therapy get all-encompassing assistance that goes beyond medical care.

Hospitals, clinics, community centers, or private firms can provide accessible counseling services. For those who are unable to attend in-person visits, teletherapy services such as video sessions and phone consultations provide easy access to counseling help. Whatever its form, getting expert counseling may make a big difference in the general health of liver disease patients and their carers.

Reliable Sources For Liver Disease Information

For patients, caregivers, and medical professionals, having access to accurate and trustworthy information on liver disease is essential in the digital era. Trusted sources are valuable resources for learning about a condition's origins, symptoms, diagnosis, available treatments, and prognosis. Those who arm themselves with reliable knowledge are better able to make choices about their care and health.

The most trustworthy information sources are medical facilities and groups that focus on liver health. Reputable hospitals, research facilities, and charitable organizations often include extensive resources on their websites, such as data sheets, articles, and instructional materials specifically designed for liver illness. Medical specialists have either written or examined these materials, guaranteeing their veracity and authenticity.

Via their official websites, government health authorities also provide reliable information about liver illness. For liver health and disease prevention, the World Health Organization (WHO), the Centers for Disease Control and Prevention (CDC), and the National Institutes of Health (NIH) provide evidence-based tools, recommendations, and data. These platforms are a reliable source of current information and advice for both patients and caregivers.

Moreover, clinical studies and scientific research papers on liver illness are published in peer-reviewed medical publications, providing insights into new therapies, diagnostic methods, and prognostic variables. While subscriptions or institutional access may be necessary to see journal articles, many journals provide free abstracts and summaries that give insightful looks at the most recent developments.

Reputable organizations online patient advocacy groups and forums may also be trustworthy resources for information and assistance. These platforms often include community forums, expert-led webinars, and carefully selected material where users can exchange stories, pose questions, and have access to resources. Participating in these groups may increase one's understanding and help one make contact with other liver disease sufferers.

When navigating the huge amount of material available on liver illness, it's crucial to assess the reliability of sources, give priority to content that is supported by evidence, and seek the advice of medical specialists for specific assistance and clarification. People may empower themselves to actively engage in their healthcare journey and advocate for their well-being by using trustworthy sources.

CHAPTER 9

Preventing Liver Disease

Prevention Strategies For Maintaining Liver Health

Maintaining liver health proactively is essential for general health. The following are some practical preventive techniques to maintain the best possible health for your liver:

1. A well-balanced diet is essential for maintaining the health of the liver. Make sure your meals are full of nutritious grains, lean meats, fruits, and veggies. Refined sweets, processed meals, and saturated fats should be consumed in moderation since they may strain the liver and aggravate fatty liver disease.

2. Moderate Alcohol drinking: One of the main causes of liver damage is excessive alcohol drinking.

Restrict your alcohol consumption to moderate amounts, which are typically one drink for women and two for men each day.

3. **Frequent Exercise:** Exercise regularly supports liver health in addition to helping one maintain a healthy weight. To lower your risk of fatty liver disease and other liver-related disorders, try to engage in moderate exercise for at least 30 minutes on most days of the week.

4. **Avoiding Hazardous Substances:** Steer away from prescription pharmaceuticals and illegal narcotics, particularly if they may cause liver damage. Before beginning any new drug or supplement, always get medical advice.

5. **Adopt Safe Sexual Behavior:** Intercourse may spread hepatitis B and C. To lower your chance of contracting viral hepatitis, practice safe sex by using

condoms and limiting the number of sexual partners you have.

6. Keep Your Weight in Check: Non-alcoholic fatty liver disease (NAFLD) and non-alcoholic steatohepatitis (NASH) are two liver illnesses that are strongly associated with obesity. You may drastically reduce your chance of getting these illnesses by keeping a healthy weight via food and exercise.

7. Keep Yourself Hydrated: Consuming enough water promotes healthy liver function and aids in the removal of toxins from the body. To keep your body and liver hydrated, try to consume eight glasses or more of water each day.

8. Get Regular Check-ups: Medical experts can monitor the condition of your liver and identify any possible problems early on with regular check-ups. Pay attention to the suggestions made by your

healthcare practitioner for regular exams and screenings, particularly if you have liver disease risk factors.

Adopting these preventative actions and choosing a healthy lifestyle will help you lower your risk of liver disease and maintain liver health over the long run.

Vaccinations For Hepatitis Viruses

Globally, viral hepatitis, especially hepatitis B and C, is a danger to liver health. Thankfully, there are vaccinations available to guard against liver damage and hepatitis infections. What you should know about hepatitis virus immunizations is as follows:

1. **Hepatitis B vaccination:** Contact with contaminated blood or body fluids may result in the transmission of the hepatitis B virus. Vaccination is very efficient in avoiding this illness. Usually, the vaccination is given in a course of three or four doses spread out over a few months. All newborns,

kids, and teenagers should have it, as should adults who are more likely to get hepatitis B, such as those who work in healthcare, have several sexual partners, or use drugs.

2. Hepatitis A Vaccine: The two main ways that hepatitis A is transmitted are via intimate contact with infected people and contaminated food or water. Children, anyone visiting areas with high hepatitis A rates, those suffering from chronic liver illness, and everyone looking for long-term protection against the virus are all advised to get the hepatitis A vaccination. Typically, the vaccination is given in two doses, separated by six months.

3. Combination vaccines: A few vaccinations provide simultaneous protection against many hepatitis viruses. For those who need protection against both viruses, the hepatitis A and hepatitis B combination vaccine, for instance, offers immunity against both hepatitis A and hepatitis B infections. This simplifies the immunization procedure.

4. Immunization Schedule: To provide the best defense against hepatitis viruses, it is important to follow the advised immunization schedule. Based on your age, medical history, and risk factors, your healthcare professional may advise you on the best time and dose for hepatitis vaccinations.

5. Vaccine Safety: There are very few adverse effects and most hepatitis vaccines are safe and well-tolerated. Pain at the injection site, a low temperature, or exhaustion are common side effects that usually go away on their own in a few days. It is uncommon for hepatitis immunizations to have serious side effects.

6. The importance of vaccination for public health cannot be overstated in the fight against hepatitis epidemics.

Healthcare professionals can dramatically lower the frequency of acute and chronic liver illness as well as stop the virus from spreading across communities by immunizing people who are at risk of contracting hepatitis.

7. Access to Vaccines: Improving vaccination accessibility is crucial to lowering the worldwide incidence of viral hepatitis, especially in impoverished areas and nations with low incomes. Expanding vaccination coverage and reaching vulnerable groups requires the implementation of public health programs, immunization campaigns, and the development of healthcare infrastructure.

We can significantly improve the chances of avoiding hepatitis infections and preserving liver health for future generations by guaranteeing universal access to hepatitis vaccinations and encouraging immunization campaigns.

Screening Recommendations For At-Risk Individuals

Improving outcomes and treating liver disease need early identification and action. Screening guidelines for those who are at risk aid in the early detection of liver diseases, when therapy is most successful. Here's a summary of the recommendations for screening groups that are at risk:

1. Hepatitis B Screening: To find out whether they have the hepatitis B virus (HBV) in their blood, those who are more likely to get the disease should be screened. Being born to a mother who has HBV, engaging in unprotected sexual activity with an infected partner, sharing needles or other drug paraphernalia, and working in healthcare environments where blood or body fluids are often handled are risk factors for contracting hepatitis B. Blood tests to find antibodies to the HBV core

antigen (anti-HBc) and the HBV surface antigen (HBsAg) may be used in screening.

2. Hepatitis C Screening: For those who are at a higher risk of coming into contact with the hepatitis C virus (HCV), screening for infection is advised. A history of injectable drug use, organ transplants or blood transfusions received before 1992, being born into an HCV-positive mother, and long-term hemodialysis are risk factors for hepatitis C. Blood tests are often used in screening to identify HCV antibodies and, if antibodies are found, follow-up testing for HCV RNA.

3. Tests for Liver Function: Liver function tests, or LFTs, are often performed to evaluate the health of the liver and identify abnormalities in liver function. LFTs evaluate a range of blood components, including proteins, enzymes, and other chemicals, which may be indicative of liver malfunction or injury. Even though LFTs are not a particular

screening tool for liver disease, unusual findings might call for more analysis and diagnostic research.

4. Imaging Studies: A variety of imaging modalities, including magnetic resonance imaging (MRI), computed tomography (CT), and ultrasound, may be used to assess the liver's structure and function and identify any anomalies or indicators of liver disease. To support diagnosis and treatment planning, these imaging modalities may enable medical professionals to see the liver, gallbladder, bile ducts, and surrounding organs.

5. Fibrosis Assessment: Non-invasive testing and imaging methods may be used to evaluate the degree of liver fibrosis (scarring) and establish the stage of liver disease in people with known or suspected liver illness. Serum-based fibrosis indicators, magnetic resonance elastography (MRE), and transient elastography (FibroScan) are some of

these assays. The evaluation of fibrosis aids in directing therapy choices and tracking the advancement of the illness over time.

6. **Screening Frequency:** Individual risk factors, underlying medical problems, and healthcare practitioner recommendations may all affect how often a patient gets screened for liver disease. For instance, routine monitoring using blood tests, imaging investigations, and liver function tests may be necessary for those with chronic hepatitis B or hepatitis C to evaluate disease activity and treatment response.

7. The significance of early identification lies in the ability to treat and intervene promptly, which may assist stop or slow the course of liver damage and enhance long-term results. The goal of screening guidelines is to find liver disorders early on when therapies have the greatest chance of averting consequences and maintaining liver function.

At-risk persons may take proactive measures to monitor their liver health, discover liver disease early, and get appropriate medical care and treatment by adhering to screening guidelines customized to their particular risk profiles. Frequent screening is essential for reducing the risk of complications from liver disease and enhancing general health.

CHAPTER 10

Living With Liver Disease

Coping Mechanisms For Managing Chronic Liver Conditions

Although having a chronic liver disease might be difficult, there are coping strategies that can guide you through the highs and lows of taking care of your health. Learning about your disease is one of the most crucial tactics. Being aware of how your liver works and how your particular ailment affects it can help you make choices regarding your treatment that are well-informed.

Creating a solid support system is a crucial additional coping method. Having individuals you can depend on for emotional support—be it friends, family, or support groups—may significantly impact your general well-being.

In addition, if you're having trouble coping, don't be afraid to get expert assistance. Guidance and emotional support may be obtained from therapists, counselors, and liver disease support groups.

It's also critical for those with chronic liver diseases to manage their stress. Stress might intensify the disease's symptoms and even hasten its course. Including stress-reduction practices in your daily routine, such as yoga, deep breathing exercises, meditation, or mindfulness, may help you manage your stress levels.

Furthermore, the management of liver disease necessitates a healthy lifestyle. This includes maintaining a healthy diet, exercising often, abstaining from alcohol and tobacco, and carefully adhering to any treatment programs or drug recommendations. Your overall health and liver health may be greatly impacted by even little changes in lifestyle behaviors.

Finally, it's critical to continue treating your disease proactively. This entails keeping a careful eye on your symptoms, scheduling regular checkups with your doctor, and standing up for yourself if you think your treatment plan needs to be modified. You may better control your liver illness and have a high quality of life by actively participating in your healthcare.

Maintaining Quality Of Life While Living With Liver Disease

Living with liver disease means having to manage your mental and physical health to maintain a great quality of life. Effective symptom management is essential for preserving quality of life. This might include using painkillers to ease discomfort, altering one's diet to enhance liver function, and changing one's way of life to put less strain on the liver.

To maintain liver function and general well-being, diet is essential. Eat a diet high in fruits, vegetables, whole grains, and lean meats to promote healthy liver function and minimize inflammation. Limiting processed foods, sweets, and saturated fats is also crucial since they put stress on the liver and aggravate symptoms.

Another crucial component of preserving the quality of life in the face of liver illness is regular exercise. Exercise may lessen weariness, elevate mood, support liver function, and help one maintain a healthy weight in addition to enhancing general fitness. To get the most advantages, try a combination of strength training, flexibility training, and cardiovascular activity.

Prioritizing mental and emotional health is crucial, in addition to physical wellness. Having a chronic disease may hurt mental health, increasing the likelihood of experiencing stress, anxiety, or depression. Joining support groups, getting treatment from mental health specialists, or learning relaxation methods may all help in managing emotional difficulties and enhancing one's general quality of life.

Keeping up social ties is essential for a high quality of life as well. Seek out chances for social connection, engage in activities you like, and maintain relationships with friends and family. Maintaining a good quality of life requires emotional support, companionship, and a feeling of belonging, all of which may be found in a robust support network.

Last but not least, keeping up with developments in liver disease research and care might inspire optimism for the future. New drugs, therapies, and treatments are always being discovered, which might be beneficial for people with liver disease. You may continue to have hope for better results and a higher standard of living in the years to come if you remain proactive and knowledgeable about your healthcare.

Hope For The Future: Advances In Liver Disease Research And Treatment

For those suffering from liver illness, new developments in the field's understanding and management provide hope. A notable advancement has been made in the creation of novel drugs and treatments for a range of liver conditions. Researchers are always looking for novel therapy alternatives to help patients get better results. These include immunosuppressants for autoimmune liver illnesses and antiviral medications for hepatitis C.

Liver transplant research is another exciting subject of study. For those suffering from acute liver failure or end-stage liver disease, liver transplantation may be a life-saving procedure. Technological developments in organ preservation, surgery, and immunosuppressive drugs have increased the number of possible donors and increased transplant success rates, providing hope to those in need of one.

Additionally, advances in comprehending the fundamental causes of liver illness are helping researchers identify possible therapeutic targets. Through the process of dissecting the intricate biology of liver illnesses, including liver cancer, cirrhosis, and nonalcoholic fatty liver disease (NAFLD), researchers are discovering novel avenues for therapy and intervention.

Along with improvements in medicine, liver illness is becoming more widely recognized and advocated for, which has raised money for studies and made patient treatment more accessible. Liver health organizations put up a great effort to increase public awareness, encourage early diagnosis and detection, and provide assistance to those who are afflicted with liver illness.

For those with liver disease, the outlook seems bright overall. Continuous progress in research, therapy, and advocacy holds promise for greater quality of life, better outcomes, and eventually a cure for many complicated disorders. Liver disease patients may look forward to a better future by being knowledgeable, proactive, and optimistic.

CONCLUSION

To sum up, liver disease is a complex issue that has a big impact on people's health, the healthcare system, and their well-being. Several important revelations have come to light throughout this investigation.

First off, the term "liver disease" refers to a wide range of illnesses, including cirrhosis, liver cancer, fatty liver disease, and viral hepatitis. The distinct etiologies, risk factors, and clinical symptoms of each subtype need specialized methods for diagnosis, treatment, and prevention.

Second, there is a significant and growing worldwide burden of liver disease, which is caused by several causes including the increased incidence of diabetes, obesity, alcohol abuse, and viral hepatitis. Disparities in the public's knowledge and education, socioeconomic determinants of health, and access to healthcare services all contribute to this burden.

Thirdly, a complete, multidisciplinary approach is necessary for efforts aimed at treating liver disease to be successful. Prioritizing lifestyle changes, hepatitis virus vaccinations, and public health initiatives aimed at risk factors including alcohol use and viral transmission should be the main focus of prevention efforts. The significance of early detection and prompt intervention emphasizes the need for routine screening, innovative diagnostic techniques, and integrated care pathways.

Furthermore, better treatment options such as medication, surgery, and liver transplantation have the potential to improve liver disease patients' prognosis and quality of life. All-encompassing strategies that take care of dietary, rehabilitative, and psychological requirements must be used in conjunction with these therapies.

Moreover, studies focused on clarifying the fundamental causes of liver illness, finding new biomarkers, and creating tailored treatments are essential for advancing this area of study.

To summarize, the fight against liver disease requires coordinated efforts on many fronts, such as clinical practice, community involvement, healthcare policy, and scientific innovation. We may work toward a future where liver disease is successfully avoided, identified early, and treated to the best of our abilities, therefore reducing its impact on people, families, and communities everywhere by encouraging cooperation and synergy between stakeholders.

THE END

www.ingramcontent.com/pod-product-compliance
Lightning Source LLC
Chambersburg PA
CBHW070312230526
45470CB00002B/839